I0500103

Do we really need someone to complete our life?

Effective home remedies for earache

How to get rid of jock itch

Health benefits of red onion

Raw food Vs cooked food which is best

Causes and dangers of low sugar level

Natural ways to treat itchy eyes

You can boost your health in just 5 minutes a day

Top 7 vitamins for women

Health problems one faces after drinking bottled water

Dangerous effects of painkillers on your health

Metabolism boosting veggies and their benefits

Foods that keep your liver happy

What happens to your body when you stop smoking

Healthy tips to redefine your jaw line

Herbs that boost your immunity

7 Foods that increases life and its quality

What makes you old and what makes you young

Incredible health benefits of oregano

Top vegetables to grow taller

Disorders related to the digestive system

9 warning signs of eating too much salt

Why you should not eat instant noodles

10 foods that help fight stomach troubles

Every woman should know about menopause

How yogurt help you to lose weight

Super foods that can cure cough

Top 5 cures for tonsillitis

Amazing health benefits of onion powder

Things to know before putting eye drops

Do you know the benefits of aspirin

DIY health tests women should take at home

Remedies for passing out intestinal gas or flatulence

what your nails say about your health

Outdoor workout tips for city people

Foods to get rid of arthritis pain

Live life on your terms

ENT Ear Nose Throat

Blood Pressure

Stretching Exercises

Stomach

Sleep

Agarbatti Dhoop

Havan

Food home made

Healthy food

Foods sold on streets in India

Reasons to drink black tea everyday

Amazing uses of whey (Left over water from paneer)

Why rest is as important as exercise

Sleeping with feet facing the door is unhealthy

Best protein shakes for muscle building

What causes weight gain after marriage?

Harmony in relationships

Happy things to do before breakfast

How to create a perfect sleep environment

What type of headache do you suffer from?

Importance of curd to your body

Foods diabetics must consume everyday

Is there a diet to increase height?

Why fermented dairy products are healthy

Proven benefits of banana

How to improve your blood

Horrible contents that is used to make fizzy drinks

Unfortunate truth of canned food

Citrus fruits the best formula to lose weight

What happens when you eat leftover foods?

Fast Food Fresh Food Packaged Food

Amazing health benefits of olives

7 things you should not do early morning

Health questions every man is afraid to ask

10 low calorie healthy foods for overweight women

Fresh herbs that make you healthier

Grandma remedies to clear sinus congestion

How emotionally mature are you

Difference between healthy and unhealthy calories

What does fiber do to your body?

7 Reasons to eat dark chocolate for the heart

Latest interesting facts about diabetes

Three most important gifts of Self Discipline you will love

7 Men's workout mistakes to avoid

Veggies that fight pancreatic cancer

Here is why you should take a walk right now

Unknown health benefits of black beans

Surprising health benefits of coriander

How your body gets energy

Did you know homeopathic medicines too have side effects?

10 genuine reasons to detox

Top liver healthy foods to eat

Why omelet is a good breakfast option

Health benefits of cow ghee

Why you should not take calcium pills

Healthy herbal teas that detoxify the body

Ayurveda Medicines

Amazing foods to increase blood platelets

Vinegar treats kidney stone Amazed Read here

Is eating in plastic container dangerous

Benefits of cabbage soup

12 ways Jeera water benefits your health

7 Signs you had a good workout

The truth about good foods and bad foods

7 Ways to unclog a stuffy nose

Top iron rich foods to include in diet

How to break a bad habit

Sleep deprivation and stress: How they are linked

Free ways to improve your health

Healthy foods that clean the colon

Health benefits of Elaichi

Amazing health benefits of red grapes

Eat these Nutrient Dense foods when you are ill and weak

Why you must take care of your brain

Be Aware: Your toothpaste can make you sick

Avoid adding these foods to your grocery cart

7 Myths about carbohydrates busted

Why drink salt water in morning

How to use a single onion in treating many common diseases

Most important meal of the day

Top herbs that prevent cancer

How gooseberry benefits health

Eight best protein snack that you can munch on

7 Things that happen to your body when you eat egg

Why exercise is better than dieting

Easy ways to cure colon cancer

Quick steps to eliminate bad breath

Is there any exercise to boost libido

Using coconut oil to detoxify

How to nourish your mind body soul

Best high antioxidant foods for women

Stop believing these nutrition myths

What happens to your body when you eat banana

How diet affects your mind

Vegetables that kill stomach fat in a week

Nutritious healthy ingredients for salad

Spices that promote weight loss

Top ten healthiest fishes you must eat

7 Reasons swimming is safe for your joints

National Cleanliness Day Why cleanliness is important

Breakfast foods for a beautiful you

What is the best lunch to avoid sleepiness?

Unique benefits of walnut

Health benefits of a Dosa

Foods which increase stomach acid for proper digestion and a ...

Hygiene mistakes that may affect your health

Simple detox ingredients that flush out toxins

Unique method may re grow hair

Treat acidity naturally with these ingredients

Health benefits of Upma

Eat these foods to get iodine in your body before it is too late

8 Amazing health benefits of salt

Health myths that you should know

Healthy foods that relieve stress

After waking up why do you feel tired?

What happens to your body after becoming a vegetarian?

How salt affects your health

What your lips say about your health

How to keep depression at bay

Ways to keep yourself happy

Why cold drinks are bad for you

8 Best liquids drink before breakfast

Hookah Myths and truth

Incredible health benefits of brown rice

Health benefits of idli sambar

Foods that kill libido

8 Home remedies for better health

Reasons why we snore in our sleep

How besan helps you lose weight

Why is it getting harder to stay healthy?

Beware: Your lipstick might have lead

5 drinks that shrink your belly

Tips to deal with menopause

15 reasons to drink milk

Which tea is good for you as per your blood group?

Benefits of sleeping with wet socks

Bitter remedies for intestinal worms

What happens when you eat bhindi regularly?

End of life; care India not among the best places to die either

10 super foods that make you happy

Natural cure for snoring

7 super foods that boost your eyesight

Ways to get rid of these fats in your body

The soup that kills cancer

Thyroid

Things that happen to your body when you lack sleep

What happens to our body when we exercise?

Best ways to boost your metabolism

7 steps to a healthy digestive system

Therapeutic benefits of aquarium therapy

How to cleanse your inside naturally

Weird mistakes we make with our teeth

7 symptoms of ulcer you should aware of

Why eggs should not be kept in the fridge

Navaratra Special Thali

Antibiotics

To de stress Chinese women live like monks

The stem plant that boosts your immunity

Simple ways to add proteins to Indian food

8 most important nutrients for good health

How can you keep your mind under control?

Ways to stay fit without gym

15 tricks to try if you want to stay healthy

Benefits you reap from vitamin D

How many times should you wash your hands?

Men feel threatened by intellectual women

10 Best health apps to get on your phone right now

10 ways to beat stress at workplace

Stretching Exercises

Blood Pressure

ENT Ear Nose Throat

Stomach

Prolonged use of sanitary napkins can put you to risk of cancer

Natural pain killers in your kichten

Health benefits of drinking water from a copper bottle or glass

Is waxing bad

What you should know about your BP

Your earphones are making you deaf slowly

Early morning water drinks that make you slim within a month

How diet affects your mind

Amazing foods to increase blood platelets

Eat these foods in winter for weight loss and warmth

Healthy reasons to eat raspberries

Amazing health benefits of sesame

Benefits of vegetable broth

10 best ways to take care of your joints

7 Horrifying facts about ckicken meat

How to improve your blood

Breakfast foods for a beautiful you

Health benefits of Upma

Vitamin B rich foods for faster hair growth

Health benefits of a Dosa

Surprising reasons to include sodium in your diet

Unexpected 7 spices that keep you warm in winter

7 Things that happen to your body when you eat egg

Stop believing these nutrition myths

Amazing health benefits of chia seeds

Yoga Sutras by Patanjali

Is distracted dining harmful

What makes siblings good?

What causes weight gain after marriage?

Happy things to do before breakfast

How to create a perfect sleep environment

What type of headache do you suffer from?

Importance of curd to your body

How to use water as medicine

Things to consider before taking pain killers

Foods diabetics must consume everyday

Is there a diet to increase height?

Why fermented dairy products are healthy

Proven benefits of banana

Horrible contents that is used to make fizzy drinks

Unfortunate truth of canned food

Citrus fruits: The best formula to lose weight

What happens when you eat leftover foods?

Fast Food Fresh Food Packaged Food

Amazing health benefits of olives

7 things you should not do early morning

Health questions every man is afraid to ask

10 low calorie healthy foods for overweight women

Fresh herbs that make you healthier

Grandma remedies to clear sinus congestion

Difference between healthy and unhealthy calories

What does fiber do to your body?

7 Reasons to eat dark chocolate for the heart

Latest interesting facts about diabetes

Three most important gifts of Self Discipline you will love

7 Men's workout mistakes to avoid

Veggies that fight pancreatic cancer

Here is why you should take a walk right now

Unknown health benefits of black beans

Surprising health benefits of coriander

How your body gets energy

Did you know homeopathic medicines too have side effects?

10 genuine reasons to detox

Top liver healthy foods to eat

Why omelets is a good breakfast option

Health benefits of cow ghee

Why you should not take calcium pills

Healthy herbal teas that detoxify the body

Ayurveda Medicines

Vinegar treats kidney stone Amazed Read here

Is eating in plastic container dangerous

Benefits of cabbage soup

12 ways jeera water benefits your health

The truth about good foods and bad foods

7 Ways to unclog a stuffy nose

Top iron rich foods to include in diet

How to break a bad habit

Sleep deprivation and stress How they are linked

Free ways to improve your health

Healthy foods that clean the colon

Health benefits of Elaichi

Amazing health benefits of red grapes

Eat these Nutrient Dense foods when you are ill and weak

Why you must take care of your brain

Be Aware: Your toothpaste can make you sick

Avoid adding these foods to your grocery cart

7 Myths about carbohydrates busted

Why drink salt water in morning

How to use a single onion in treating many common diseases...

Most important meal of the day

Top herbs that prevent cancer

How gooseberry benefits health

Eight best protein snack that you can munch on

Why exercise is better than dieting

Easy ways to cure colon cancer

Quick steps to eliminate bad breath

Is there any exercise to boost libido

How to clean up your diet

Using coconut oil to detoxify

Simple detox ingredients that flush out toxins

How to nourish your mind body soul

Best high antioxidant foods for women

Vegetables that kill stomach fat in a week

Nutritious healthy ingredients for salad

Life is all about your mind and heart

How beautiful is your mind

Top ten healthiest fishes you must eat

7 Reasons swimming is safe for your joints

What is the best lunch to avoid sleepiness?

Unique benefits of walnut

Foods not to eat in the morning

Jumping cures depression, want to know how

Hygiene mistakes that may affect your health

Foods which increase stomach acid for proper digestion and a ...

Unique method may regrow hair

Treat acidity naturally with these ingredients

Eat these foods to get iodine in your body before it is too late

8 Amazing health benefits of salt

Health myths that you should know

Healthy foods that relieve stress

After waking up why do you feel tired?

What happens to your body after becoming a vegetarian?

What your lips say about your health

Why cold drinks are bad for you

8 Best liquids drink before breakfast

Hookah Myths and truth

Incredible health benefits of brown rice

Health benefits of idli sambar

Foods that kill libido

8 Home remedies for better health

Reasons why we snore in our sleep

How besan helps you lose weight

Why is it getting harder to stay healthy?

Beware your lipstick might have lead

5 drinks that shrink your belly

Tips to deal with menopause

15 reasons to drink milk

Which tea is good for you as per your blood group?

Benefits of sleeping with wet socks

What is the tongue telling you about your health?

Foods that melt your love handles

Can you lose weight during sleep?

Best ways to clear your toxins in 7days

What does jogging do to your brain

Simple ways smokers can purify their lungs

10 ways to improve your personal hygiene

Look at your feet to check if you are healthy

Benefits of hydrotherapy

8 Vegetables that you should be juicing

Exercise you can do in bed every morning

Healthy foods that soothe you sore muscles

Benefits of walking without shoes

Why chicken nuggets are bad for health

Ladies alert Learn how love making benefits you

Healthy foods to kill stress

Indian food that are weight loss friendly

Know what a 30 minute 40 minute 60 minute walk is doing to you

Avoid these unhealthy mistakes in a bathroom

Simple tricks to relax your mind body

Myths about spicy food

An exercise for lower back pain

7 Healthier alternatives to sugar

Why chose a workout that is safe for joints

What happens to your body when you eat curd

Easy ways to cure liver disease

Side effects of healthy nutritious food

Incredible health benefits of red banana

Amazing health benefits of Amla soaked honey

Strange health benefits of snacking

Health benefits of social life

Amazing health benefits of spring onion

It is time to add these 2016 Super foods to your diet

Does the TV make you gain weight?

Are shopping and happiness linked?

Remedies to reduce alcohol craving

Types of fish that are, unhealthy to eat

10 Unique ways to meditate

Foods every married man must add to his diet

Why heart patients should avoid sitting too much

Top kidney cleansing herbs and drinks

Natural ways to treat acidity

Amazing super foods to beat stress and anxiety

Ways to include raw veggies in your diet

Healthy veggies that you are avoiding

Why it is okay to have a little belly fat

Junk foods that are actually healthy and good for you

Bad food combination that make you sick

Be aware These daily products harm the thyroid gland

8 Healthy habits that are, extremely unhealthy

Foods that cleanse intestines and aid weight loss

Health benefits of Moong dal sprouts: 9 Unknown nutrition facts

A magical combo Warm milk turmeric Haldi benefits on yo ...

Foods to help you sleep

Which food is best to eat according to your age

10 health benefits of potato juice

How cloves benefit your health

How mobile radiation effects health

Do you know what happens to your body when you are lazy

8 body parts that you are not using

Want to lose weight follow banana diet

Unknown health benefits of papaya leaves

Health benefits of massaging feet before bedtime

How to improve your digestive system naturally

10 miraculous benefits of eating cloves daily

Use turmeric as a natural alternative for these drugs

health benefis of drinking warm milk honey

10 common walking mistakes to avoid

Reasons to drink aloa vera juice every day

Morning rituals to supercharge your metabolism

8 roots you should eat everyday

Simple tips to get rid of hiccups instantly

unknown healthy benefits of papaya seed

Secrets healthy India women follow

what PMS does to a woman every month

7 ways pumpkin juice benefits your health

Ways breathing right can improve your body

Strange ways Sun affects your body

The healing powers of fruits

Healthy breakfast recipes for your

school going kids

7 simple but life changing health decisions

Do you know what happens when you pop in pills

How many times should you wash your hands

How can you keep your mind under control

8 most important nutrients for good health

To de stress Chinese women live like monks

Why eggs should not be kept in the fridge

7 symptoms of ulcer you should aware of

Weird mistakes we make with our teeth

Therapeutic benefits of aquarium

therapy

What happens to our body when we exercise

Things that happen to your body when you lack sleep

7 super foods that boost your eyesight

Natural cure for snoring

10 super foods that make you happy

What happens when you eat Bhindi regularly

Can raw food cure diabetes

Health benefits of Chana Dal

Does too much of salt damage your liver

Know why you should eat fruits in the first meal of the day

Health benefits of drinking butter milk in summer

Foods that increase bone strength

Remedies to reduce alcohol craving

Why chicken nuggets are bad for health

Benifits of sleeping with wet socks

Types of fish that are unhealthy to eat

Foods every married man must add to his diet

Vitamin B rich foods for faster hair growth

Eat these foods in winter for weight loss and warmth

Why heart patients should avoid sitting too much

How to target belly fat depending on its type

Health hizards of using mobile phones

Top kidney cleansing herbs and drinks

What does jogging do to your brain

Natural ways to treat acidity

Amazing super foods to beat stress and anxiety

How emotionally mature are you

aapo deepo bhava be a light unto your self

Life is all about your mind and heart

10 Unique ways to meditate

Ways to include raw veggies in your diet

Importance of curd to your body

Low carb snacks to satisfy hunger

How your father s diet affects your health

Healthy veggies that you are avoiding

7 Things that happen to your body when you eat egg

Early morning water drinks that make you slim within a month

Is distracted dining harmful

Bad food combination that make you sick

Why it is okay to have a little belly fat

Can you lose weight during sleep

Sleep deprivation and stress How they are linked

Junk foods that are actually healthy and good for you

Best high antioxidant foods for women

Be aware These daily products harm the thyroid gland

8 Healthy habits that are extremely unhealthy

Help others and beat your stress level

Foods that cleanse intestines and aid weight loss

Indian food that are weight loss friendly

10 Foods fashion models eat to stay slim

A magical combo Warm milk turmeric Haldi benefits on your...

Foods to help you sleep

10 ways to improve your personal hygiene

10 best ways to take care of your joints

Which food is best to eat according to your age

iron rich foods to combat anaemia

10 health benefits of potato juice

how cloves benefit your health

Bed time drinks to melt belly fat in 15 days

How mobile radiation effects health

Do you know what happens to your body when you are lazy

Breaking Myths Is curd bad for your

health

Want to lose weight follow banana diet

8 body parts that you are not using

Amazing health benefits of chia seeds

Foods that kill libido

Avoid these unhealthy mistakes in a bathroom

Try this one drink to avoid cancer

Unknown health benefits of papaya leaves

Health benefits of massaging feet before bedtime

How to improve your digestive system naturally

4 types of people who must avoid ginger

10 miraculous benefits of eating cloves daily

Use turmeric as a natural alternative

for these drugs

Health benefits of drinking warm milk
honey

10 common walking mistakes to avoid

Reasons to drink aloe Vera juice every
day

Morning rituals to supercharge your
metabolism

New food safety norms

Beware Your lipstick might have lead

Healthy Food

Alcoholic

10 miraculous benefits of eating cloves
daily

Use turmeric as a natural alternative
for these drugs

Health benefits of drinking warm milk
honey

10 common walking mistakes to avoid

Reasons to drink aloe Vera juice every day

Morning rituals to supercharge your metabolism

New food safety norms

Beware Your lipstick might have lead

Healthy Food

Alcoholic

Most important meal of the day

Simple ways smokers can purify their lungs

What happens when you eat bhindi regularly

Ladies alert Learn how love making benefits you

10 super foods that make you happy

Look at your feet to check if your

healthy

Natural cure for snoring

How to use water as medicine

7 super foods that boost your eyesight

Ways to get rid of these fats in your body

The soup that kills cancer

Things that happen to your body when you lack sleep

What happens to our body when we exercise

Spices that promote weight loss

what type of headache do you suffer from

Best ways to boost your metabolism

7 steps to a healthy digestive system

Therapeutic benefits of aquarium therapy

8 Home remedies for better health

Foods diabetics must consume everyday

Opting for natural ...

How to cleanse your inside naturally

Weird mistakes we make with our teeth

7 symptoms of ulcer you should aware of

What is the tongue telling you about your health

why eggs should not be kept in the fridge

5 drinks that shrink your belly

vegetables that kill stomach fat in a week

The stem plant that boosts your immunity

Horrible contents that is used to make fizzy drinks

How to improve your blood

Simple ways to add proteins to Indian food

8 most important nutrients for good health

How can you keep your mind under control

How besan helps you lose weight

Ways to stay fit without gym

food that keeps your liver happy

15 tricks to try if you want to stay healthy

Why is it getting harder to stay healthy

Healthy foods to kill stress

Benefits you reap from vitamin D

How many times should you wash your hands

Men feel threatened by intellectual

women

Benefits of vegetable broth

Do you know what happens when you pop in pills

Surprising reasons to include sodium in your diet

Healthy things to do on a holiday

Real reasons why you can not lose weight

Why exercise is better than dieting

7 detoxifying super foods

7 simple but life changing health decisions

Follow this diet to improve blood count

Tips to lower blood pressure naturally

7 ways to improve hygiene

Why do we crave for junk food

Healthy ways to stay awake at night

Follow these remedies if you hate flossing

How to clean up your diet

Top 5 fat burning super food

Exercises that tone your legs in a week

Healthy breakfast recipes for your school going kids

Unique method may re grow lost hair

Top five alkaline fruits

The healing powers of fruits

Strange ways Sun affects your body

Ways breathing right can improve your body

Health benefits of hugs and kisses

Do you know reason behind your body pain

Build your immunity in 7 days

7 ways pumpkin juice benefits your

health

Reasons why we snore in our sleep

Strange uses of these daily medication

What PMS does to a woman every month

What does fiber do to your body

Why are cigarettes so addictive

The true meaning of education

Healthy foods that become dangerous

Amazing health benefits of sesame

Reasons to eat almonds everyday

Health tips for married women on Karva Chauth

Secrets healthy India women follow

Citrus fruits The best formula to lose weight

Unique benefits of walnut

Unknown healthy benefits of papaya

seed

Using coconut oil to detoxify

Best ways to clear your toxins in 7days

Crazy ways to burn calories through out the day

Why fermented dairy products are healthy

10 foods that heal a broken heart

Simple tips to get rid of hiccups instantly

Best protein shakes for muscle building

Reasons of your fat belly you don't know

8 roots you should eat everyday

Want to look younger call your dentist

Weight loss lies myths we blindly believe in

Amazing health benefits of eating garlic

Natural ways to increase white blood cells

Amazing health benefits of peanut oil

The ugly truth about Trans fats in your packet of chips

Water Vs Fruit juice which is better

Know how chewing gum is bad for you

Super veggies for a healthy you

Almonds: A handful of goodness

Herbal remedies to treat stomach ache

Why you don't need dairy

Harmful foods doctors advise not to consume

Are you eating according to your zodiac sign

How anti aging super foods can work wonders for you

Mustard oil can help you stay healthy

Iron rich food to include in your diet

Health benefits of water melon juice with pepper

9 habits of fit women

Health benefits of Hing

Why warming up is crucial

8 physical effect of sleep deprivation

10 Ageing myths that no one tells you

Reasons why women should lift weights

Health benefits of dal rice

Diseases that are caused by nutritional deficiencies

Reasons to eat 3 bananas a day

Best foods that reduce gas and bloating

Side effects of wearing contact lenses

Side effects of injecting steroids in the body

World Kidney Day: Symptoms of

chronic Kidney /Renal disease

World Kidney Day: Beat kidney stones with these amazing home remedies

World Kidney Day: Natural juices to flush out kidney stone

Health benefits of Cucumber water: Cheers to the summer

Disturbing facts about soda

Natural Probiotic foods to keep your gut happy and healthy

Vegetarian food beneficial but balanced diet is key to health

House hold items that are so unhealthy to touch

Change your cooking oil every three months even doctors say so

Amazing health benefits of lemon grass

Dear women try these tips for a stress free life

Ox toxin: Know all that you need to know about the love hormon

High protein vegetarian food sources

Anti- ageing foods you need to include in diet

Go shopping if you want a longer life

Ways figs can be used to treat leg and back pain

10 Super foods that clean up your intestines

Health benefits of riding a cycle to work

Interesting facts to know about the best time to eat some foods

Pre workout meals to take before you hit the gym

How to remove pesticides from your vegetables

6 Potentially fatal diseases that women need to care about

Easy ways to remove phlegm and clear lung

Parents! Stop using Smartphone at dinner table

7 Ways to add yoghurt in your diet

This drink will cleanse your liver fast

How much a raw cucumber with meals

Herbal teas that cure sore throat

Touch your fingers to let your body heal you

Indian food habits that are healthy

This remedy cures hypertension and cholesterol

Do you know side effects of drinking too much tea

Important medical tests women should take up

How skipping breakfast leads to weight gain & diabetes

Drink this before making love...

Amazing health benefits of barley

Eating late at night can lead you to THIS disorder

Surprising health benefits of grapes

Do you know the 13 health benefits of black pepper corns?

Drink this to burn belly fat in 5 days

Amazing health benefits of Almond oil

Symptoms of down syndrome

The easiest way to fall asleep

Best Ayurveda remedies to treat PCOS

This breakfast helps lose a kilo a month

Four best ways how to shine like a diamond

Detoxifying veggies to include in your diet

This remedy cures hypertension and

cholesterol

Do you know side effects of drinking too much tea

Important medical tests women should take up

How skipping breakfast leads to weight gain & diabetes

Drink this before making love...

Amazing health benefits of barley

Eating late at night can lead you to THIS disorder

Surprising health benefits of grapes

Do you know the 13 health benefits of black pepper corns?

Drink this to burn belly fat in 5 days

Amazing health benefits of Almond oil

Symptoms of down syndrome

The easiest way to fall asleep

Best Ayurveda remedies to treat PCOS

This breakfast helps lose a kilo a month

Four best ways how to shine like a diamond

Detoxifying veggies to include in your diet

51 Foods America gave to the world

7 Secret herbs for tooth pain relief

Unknown side affects of lemon juice

World Tuberculosis Day: Facts about tuberculosis

Try this remedy for gall stone

Homemade recipes to treat urinary track infection

How Holi colors affect our health

How to get rid of stomach acid naturally

Quick remedies for tired and itchy eyes

Reasons to have lentils every day

5 secret tips for a healthy life style

Workout to increase your flexibility

A herb that cures more than 25 disorder

Health benefits of Argon oil

Wall-Sits: Tone your legs in 5 Minutes

Ways your relationship could affect your health

What you should eat for breakfast if you want to lose weight

Herbal remedies to treat digestive problem

Unknown health benefits of radish

Why raising a cat is healthy

Unknown health benefits of black beans

Why you should consume proteins

10 Healthy spices that heart patients can eat

Ayurvedic remedies for burping

Best natural antibiotics to use

What you should know about Cervical Cancer

14 things you need to know about OCD

8 Plants to keep in your bedroom for better sleep

8 Reasons to eat more lentils this summer

Beware of abnormal blood clots

Top 10 Vegetarian Protein sources

Foods that keep the kidneys happy

10 Potent home remedies to eliminate root canal pain

How fiber rich food saves your life

15 Sleep hacks for a sound sleep

10 cool ways to beat the heat in April

Herbal ways to cleans liver

7 foods and medication you should not mix

Positive calm: The secret to inner peace

Learn these 4 secrets of Chanakya for a happier life

10 Best Health Apps for Women

5 Medical Check ups to test before getting married

10 Foods we eat at wrong hours That are harming our body

Simple steps to keep your lungs happy

Know how stressed you are in just under 2 seconds

This mixture work like cough syrup

Tips for Indians to prevent diabetes

Tips to stay healthy in Indian climate

10 Preventive measures to avoid heat stroke

Signs of high acid levels in your body

Photographer reveals how much online images are photoshoped

10 things you should never do after a heart attack

Herbal ways to cleans liver

7 foods and medication you should not mix

Positive calm: The secret to inner peace

Learn these 4 secrets of Chanakya for a happier life

10 Best Health Apps for Women

5 Medical Check ups to test before getting married

10 Foods we eat at wrong hours That are harming our body

Simple steps to keep your lungs happy

Know how stressed you are in just under 2 seconds

This mixture work like cough syrup

Tips for Indians to prevent diabetes

Tips to stay healthy in Indian climate

10 Preventive measures to avoid heat stroke

Signs of high acid levels in your body

Photographer reveals how much online images are photoshoped

10 things you should never do after a heart attack

Nutritious foods that fight aging

10 Health benefits of drinking mint water in summer

Try this Evening Cleansing Juice

7 Effective ways to tone your arms

This one dry fruit helps you fight depression

7 Foods you must eat after a morning

run

8 Affordable & healthy fruits and vegetables

DIY: Effective homemade mouthwash

Bhindi + Water = No diabetes cholesterol

5 Amazing DIY ginger remedies to cure diarrhea

7 Ways your regular lifestyle habits can kill you

How to challenge your whole system

What body building steroids do to you

Turmeric juice cures depression

A soup that boots immunity

8 simple ways to relax your body in office

7 foods that are instigating your migraine headache

How to keep your body tight

Home remedies to cure kidney stones without surgery

Foods to eat for dinner to avoid summer heat

Drink warm water this summer

This magical oil treats Hypothyroidism

A drink that keeps your heart happy

Natural Cures to heal wounds

8 Affordable healthy fruits and vegetables

DIY Effective homemade mouthwash

10 Alkaline foods that prevent diseases

10 foods to have in dinner for better digestion

7 ways to cool your body in summer

World Hemophilia Day: Useful tips for Hemophilia survivors

Mixing these 3 ingredients in your morning tea would boost weight loss

10 Kitchen ingredients that treat cold cough

Wearing underwear at night is good or bad for health
Tips to help cope with chronic pain and depression

Do this if you are suffering from pain

Unknown health benefits of Rasam

What kind of parent you are according to your zodiac sign

Find out what wedding month says

about your relationship

5 Unhealthy toppings found on a pizza

A Yoga pose that heals many organs

Homemade cough syrup recipe for instant relief

Can too much exercise make you less fertile

7 things that lead to a liver failure

Reset your liver in 72 hours

10 Exercises women can do to make their back stronger

Summer safety How to get more water in your body

Get rid of that summer cold in 7 magical ways

One food no one knew can cure diabetes completely

How Earth affects your lifespan

Things to remember before going for a surgery

10 Best North Indian foods that won t make you fat

What happens when you drink turmeric water

Ways to feel good even without meditation

The many health benefits of alcohol when drunk moderation

3D imaging technique to precisely spot deadly lung disease

2 Best Ayurvedic recipes for weight loss

What happens when you drink turmeric water

Ways to feel good even without meditation

The many health benefits of alcohol when drunk in moderation

What happens to your body if you drink pepper water

Diet Vs Exercise: Which is better?
Can diabetes be prevented if you refrain from sweets

World Malaria Day: Facts about Malaria

How to keep your mind calm and stress free

Bitter ingredients that cure a headache & cold

7 remedies to treat chafing in summer

Ways to treat common skin problems in summer

What happens when you eat banana stem

5 reasons to eat potato/ aloo skin

10 risk factors of Hypothyroidism

The amazing health benefits of medical clay

This simple yoga pose rejuvenates your system

9 things that happen to you if you are overweight

Traditional healthy coolants to shun the summer heat

Importance of minerals for our body

9 foods to stay away from if you have joint pains

Major causes of weakness in legs

International Dance Day: Can Dance prevent depression

7 signs that you have parasites in your body

8 reasons that cause depression

Health benefits of shrimp

10 risk factors of Hypothyroidism

The amazing health benefits of medical clay

This simple yoga pose rejuvenates your system

What happens when you perform chakrasana

7 best no equipment workouts

7 Common herbs that boost brain health

Cucumber lemon and mint leaves Drink for weight loss

Must know Reasons to sleep on your left side

How does alcohol help body

10 foods that give natural Sun protection

What destroys your immunity

Try the banana tea

Importance of anesthesia in surgery

10 scents you need to sniff to benefit Good health

8 home made remedies that help you

stop drinking naturally

Natural remedies to get rid of piles pain

One kitchen ingredient that treats piles in 24 hrs

Are mangoes fattening or good for health

Drink this juice if you have asthma

Avoid these foods if you have asthma

3 powerful yogasana tips for asthma relief

Try this strange homemade remedy for body pain

Best diet plan for weight gain

What happens when you eat garlic and Honey for 7 days

Home remedies to cure ear pain

What is a Mono diet

8 home remedies to get relief from heal

pain naturally

Why boiled eggs are the best lunch

Why you should not follow a detox diet

Health benefits of fish pose

No health hazards due to radiation
from mobile towers: Government